HEARTBURN
TREATMENT GUIDE

HeartBurn Treatment Guide

Understanding The Causes of Heartburn And
Alleviating Heartburn Symptoms Within 14 Days

Jake Kennedy

TABLE OF CONTENT

THE CAUSES OF HEARTBURNS

Heartburns are a result when there is an excessive stomach acid leakage into the esophagus or lower throat. Acid reflux, which means that when the acid is flowing back, is a common medical tern used to explain a situation where your stomach acid flows back from the stomach of a patient to the esophagus.

This is an extremely difficult situation to deal with and would disrupt the life of the sufferer, especially those who suffer from the frequent symptoms of this troublesome illness. The patient would need to bear with a constant feeling of uneasiness and pain while they eat and drink.

Sleeping would be very difficult because the pain would get even worse when you lie down. Most people struggle with this condition because of their poor eating habits while some suffer due to their genetics.

The thing that causes heartburns are when the lower esophageal sphincter (LES) between your stomach and esophagus doesn't close up appropriately, leading to extreme damage to the esophagus. The LES is very sensitive to a lot of food and this makes it wobbly.

The food that are the biggest culprits in causing heartburns include acidic food like oranges, sweet food like chocolates and spicy food like enchiladas.

Besides these, there are also other factors which can make you develop gastroesophageal disorders. The overconsumption of alcohol or tobacco could also cause the LES to not close properly, bringing up this condition.

Factors like obesity or pregnancy also play a part. They put pressure or weight onto the stomach and causes the food that you consume to flow back. When there is an excessive amount of acid out of the stomach, it further triggers heartburn.

Daily stress and tension could also be a factor of the over-stimulation of gastric acid. As such, patients who are going through this situation would need to make certain changes in their eating habits and lifestyle.

Don't eat meal portions which are too large. Don't eat food with are full of fat and calories as well.

People who don't have an exercise routine and are always stressed out would also need to be aware. This causes a problem for your digestive system. If you want to stop the heartburn problems, you should look to stop smoking, eating fatty and spicy foods, eat smaller portion of meals and manage stress better.

If your heartburns go untreated, it would lead to even more severe disease like stomach ulcers and even cancers. We would discuss more about this in the following chapters.

If you are looking to cure or prevent heartburns, take time to slowly read this book and understand its content. It would do a great deal of help for your health.

THE SIGNS OF HEARTBURNS

In the previous chapter, I explained that when acids in your stomach raise the food pipe, it leads to heartburn. This is a digestive problem. When people hear that it is called as "heartburn", they automatically think that it is a heart problem.

Another name for heartburn is esophageal disorder and it is a burning sensation in your esophagus. The pain from heartburn could also be felt in your upper abdomen and chest area.

Generally, there are three main causes of heartburn. They include poor sleeping postures, bad food habits and wearing clothes which are overly tight. You can prevent heartburn from happening or lessening the intensity by following certain simple rules related to sleeping, food and clothing.

If one is suffering from heartburn, you have to be very careful. This is because many times, heartburn is said to be the cause of pain which impends a heart attack. To treat heartburns, it could be treated using either medication or surgery.

Medical treatment starts with antacids. They are taken as either tablet form or liquid form. They are easily available at all pharmacy and it is incredibly effective when you have mild heartburns.

However, antacids may not work if you have stronger cases of heartburn. To deal with the milder form, use H2 antagonist. H2 antagonist is a type of medication which reduces the flow and quantity of the acids in your stomach.

However, this medication isn't as popular as proton pump inhibitors have completely replaced this form of medication.

Proton pump treatment is normally prescribed to patients who are not responding to antacids or acid blockers. The principle of this medication is such; it would block the proteins and disables them. These proteins control the pH mechanism of your stomach.

Once it has achieved them, the medication would have an effect on your stomach and wouldn't let the acid from inflicting further damage on your digestion.

These inhibitors control acid from forming on your stomach and reduce the chances of heartburn. Generally, proton pump inhibitors are the most widely accepted form of medication available.

However, you would need to consult your physician first before any such medication. Most medical practitioners greatly recommend controlling your food intake while treatment is being performed.

From experience, those patients who have controlled their diet respond better to medication compared to those who have no control over their diet.

If medication doesn't work, doctor would prescribe surgery. However, this is often when you condition is very severe.

DIFFERENT TYPES OF HEARTBURNS

There are various types of heartburns, depending on several factors. This includes the cause of your heartburn and the severity of the condition.

Therefore, before you seek the appropriate treatment for this painful condition, you should know what type of heartburns that you face. Among the most common types of heartburns include:

- **Pregnancy Heartburns** - There is a possibility that pregnancy could bring about heartburn. However, pregnant mothers need not worry because these heartburn symptoms would go away when the infant is born.

During the final few months of the pregnancy, there is increased pressure on the stomach. This decelerates the digestive system and would cause the acid to stay in their stomach for a long period.

This would increase the chances of the digestive acids flowing back from the stomach to the esophagus which causes heartburns.

- **Gastro Esophageal Reflux Disease (GERD)** - This is a condition which is also known as Acid Reflux. It is the most serious and painful form of heartburns. GERB is a sign that there is a severe problem which is more than normal heartburn. If the patient suffers from heartburns more than once a week for several hours/days, there is an increased chance that you are suffering from GERD.

This isn't just a simple heartburn. If it isn't treated on time, it would lead to further chronic health problems like asthma, gingivitis, wheezing etc.

- **Summer Heartburns** - Summer is a great season to be in. Most of us consume many great foods like cheese sandwich and French fries.

  As such, this is also an increased possibility of heartburns. The increased high temperature together with the unhealthy diet means that the chances of your heartburn attacks are much higher.

  However, during the summer, you should stay away from acidic food and have lighter meals which are easy to digest.

- **Night Time Heartburn** - This is perhaps the worst kind of heartburns. Most heartburn attacks happen during the day and it would thus be easier to deal with them by medication or simply resting.

Night time heartburn attacks the patient at night when their body is relaxed and not ready to handle such pain and discomfort.

- **Chronic Heartburns** - These are the most severe and occur a few times a week (twice or thrice).

  As such frequent attacks of heartburn are a warning of more serious diseases; you need to ensure that you are properly examined by a specialist to know the reason behind your chronic heartburns.

Knowing the heartburn type that you are suffering from makes it easier to find for a treatment.

If you want to know how to deal with these conditions, read on to the next chapters. I would show you how to better understand your heartburn problems and how to treat them well.

METHODS OF ALLEVIATING HEARTBURNS

Anyone who has experienced heartburn would know how painful and unpleasant the burning sensation is. The pain in the esophagus happens when there is excessive stomach acid. However, you can easily take certain steps to alleviate this distressing condition to a great extent.

To overcome this, the best way is to look for the causes beforehand and then decide what steps to take to deal with this problem.

In the earlier chapters, I have explained that heartburns occur when there is an excessive stomach acid. This results in irritation in the esophagus and happens when the Lower Esophageal Sphincter (LES) are not sealed or closed properly.

Generally, there are two main reasons for this condition. The first major reason is when you overeat and cause to fill up your stomach excessively.

As such, the method of alleviating heartburn is to simply stop eating too much. Even if you have a dining table full of extremely delicious food, learn to limit yourself. Limiting yourself to only a moderate meal portions would help you better control your heartburn condition.

Another main reason which leads to heartburn is having too much weight or pressure over the stomach. This is especially common among pregnant mother or obese people.

To deal with this condition for pregnant ladies, a good method of controlling heartburn is to practice good posture, use a comfortable pillow and avoid sleeping immediately after meals. These are some common methods for pregnant women to reduce the discomfort.

Ideally, you should go to bed only 2-3 hours after eating. Most pregnant women complain about heartburn during their pregnancy but don't worry. It would go away after the baby is born. The symptoms would go away.

In the case of obesity, the only method of controlling heartburn situation is to lose weight. The excess weight on your stomach is the one that causes discomfort.

Those who have heartburn should avoid certain food. This includes chocolate, citrus fruits, mustard, tomatoes, juice, soda, coffee and vinegar. Other food which are oily and friend should also be avoided as they are filled with higher fat content. This leads to heartburn and blockage on your stomach.

Instead, you should look to make some changes in your daily lifestyle habits. This helps alleviate the pain and discomfort of heartburns. As you follow a good exercise and dieting program, you can improve your heartburn condition quickly.

Besides that, look to eat certain food like chamomile, aloe vera, tea and raw potatoes.

One thing that you should avoid is smoking. Smoking is a major cause of painful heartburn bouts at it stimulates the production of acid in your stomach.

Besides that, stress would also make your condition worse. Therefore, along with eating well, exercising regularly and quit smoking; look to also deal with your stress better. These lifestyle modifications could make a great difference in the life of a heartburn patient.

PERSISTENT HEARTBURNS

One of the worst forms of heartburns is persistent heartburn. They are very painful and would attack the patient a few times a week.

The common symptom of this condition includes swallowing difficulties, sore throat, chest pain and regular coughing. In more severe situations, the food would get back to the mouth even after you have swallowed.

As such, it is very important to seek medical guidance as quickly as possible. If you don't check for this situation, it could lead to even more serious complication.

When acid flows back to the esophagus, it would lead to even more serious damage. If constant heartburn isn't treated properly, it would lead to other diseases.

If your constant heartburn isn't treated on time, it would lead to even more serious diseases like ulcers in your esophagus or stricture. This implies that the esophageal slims or narrows after a certain stage.

Perhaps the worst case would be Barrett's esophagus which could even result in esophageal cancer.

However, there are certain methods that could help with the occurrence of such heartburn symptoms. Remember to do it if your heartburn attacks a few times a week. Failure to do it would severely undermine your health.

A specialist should be able to assess your condition and opt for the right actions. Major lifestyle changes are also very important in dealing with these persistent heartburns. To start, consider what you eat. This is similar to regular heartburns but you need to be more thorough about what you eat.

Consider what you eat immediately prior to having those heartburn attacks and slowly eliminate it from your meal plan. Besides that, watch out for the beverages that you drink. For example, if you have bouts of heartburn immediately after eating French fries, eliminate it from your diet.

Besides that, you should also eat more frequent meals instead of large meals because when your stomach is too full, there is increased likelihood of acid entering the esophagus.

You should also drink a lot of water as it is healthy and acts as a natural neutralizer for acids. You should also stop wearing tight-fitting clothes as it is a common cause of heartburn.

The changes in your life are similar to regular heartburns. This includes dietary changes, stress management and regular exercise.

However, if those symptoms still persist, the doctor would need to do a more thorough examination on you. They would give you the required medication and advice. Among the medication which could treat this problem include

Tagamet, H2 Blockers, Prevacid and Nexium.

NATURAL TREATMENTS TO DEAL WITH HEARTBURNS

Heartburn is a common medical condition associated with your digestive system. This happens when stomach acid flows back to your esophagus and causes a burning sensation under your sternum and breastbone. This varies from mild and irregular to serious and constant.

Heartburns are classified into its various forms depending on its severity. Chronic heartburns are a sign that there are some serious problems like hiatal hernia, peptic ulcer and gastritis. Luckily, there is an abundant of treatments available to deal with heartburns.

Among the possible treatments include Mylant, Maalax and Riopan. However, it should be clear that they only lessen the pain temporarily and doesn't provide a lasting healing effect.

The most important and effective steps when dealing with this problem is to make some major changes in your lifestyle.

Among the things to avoid when wanting to relieve yourself of painful symptoms of heartburns include alcohol, fatty food, spicy food and junk food. This avoidance would help lower the acidic level in your body to ensure that your body functions better.

Besides that, you should avoid sleeping immediately after you eat. Ideally, one should go to bed only three to four hours after their last meal.

Taking smaller meals more frequently instead of taking three big meals gives your body sufficient time for your body to digest the food. Additionally, going for walks after your meals would also help alleviate the discomfort in your stomach.

Ginger is very good to treat this condition. You can take either ginger tea, ginger tablets or even in its raw form. Besides this, you could also take chamomile, fennel tea and aloe vera juice to ease your heartburn.

Taking cumin seeds would also help speed up your digestive system. Simply take those cumin seeds together with a glass of water or with an apple after your meals.

Drinking plenty of water is also a natural treatment. Water, if consumed in the right amount, helps to charge up the metabolic rate and purifies your body. This inevitably helps your digestion.

Simple and light exercises are tremendous in helping to relieve you from this problem. Even a few minutes of moderate physical activities like walking, stretching or jogging could help improve your digestive system. It would also improve your circulation and digestive muscle movement.

All these natural treatments may seem simple, but it goes a long way towards alleviating the burning, choking and chest pain which are caused by heartburn. Besides that, you would also feel much better physically and mentally.

DRINKING HERBAL TEA TO CURE HEARTBURNS

For thousands of years, tea has been used to soothe a variety of different health problems. According to findings, tea is the most consumed beverage in the world, apart for water. Those who are looking for a natural heartburn herbal remedy could look for a good choice in herbal teas.

Certain teas like green, red and black teas contain certain polyphenols which acts as an antioxidant. It helps to protect your body from free-radical damage.

Polyphenols found in your tea is shown to provide anti-cancer properties, through various studies. The same studies also proved that drinking a few cups of tea a day would reduce your risk of gastric and esophageal cancer.

However, not all teas are the same. These teas leaves from black, red and green teas come from a form of warm-weather evergreen tree known as Camellia Sinensis. However, what is considered as herbal teas doesn't come from such a tree at all.

As a matter of fact, herbal teas are not really tea but are simply infusions known as "tisane". They are made from various flowers, herbs, roots and other plant parts. Although tisane doesn't contain as much polyphenols as true tea, it could be very beneficial in many ways.

When looking at how to remove heartburns, there are some herbal teas which are more advantageous in easing heartburn symptoms, gastrointestinal disorders and acid reflux, compared to others.

Besides that, some tea would even aggravate those conditions rather than relieving them. As such, you must choose your herbal tea remedy properly. If you are looking for a herbal tea to relieve heartburn symptoms, here a few herbal tea to consider.

❖ Marshmallow Tea

These aren't those fluffy snacks that you roast over the fire. In such a case, it is the root which is used in herbal medicinal products. When you take them internally, like in tea, marshmallow is able to ease bladder infections.

They would also coat and sooth the gastrointestinal tract, easy respiratory problems and promote the healing of the urinary tract. It is easily purchase as a topical formula, used on burns, inflammatory skin disorders and scrapes.

❖ Chamomile Tea

This is perhaps the most popular herbal tea to treat many health concerns like heartburn, anxiety, sleep disturbances and indigestion.

It would help relieve the irritated or inflamed mucus membranes of your digestive tract and promote a normal digestion process. When used topically, it would promote the healing of certain minor skin irritations and scrapes.

However, care should be taken when you take this tea. Some people have certain reactions to this.

❖ Peppermint Tea

The mint leaves, which are used to brew amazing refreshing herbal tea, contain no caffeine. There are mixed reports on whether to use peppermint when one is suffering from heartburn or acid reflux.

In many cases, it would ease your stomach and digestive problem. The peppermint oil would stimulate the flow of bile to your stomach. This helps relieve gas pains, settle stomach problems and calm heartburn.

On the other hand, research has proved that drinking peppermint or other strongly spiced tea could actually cause the LES to relax more and this results in additional acid reflux.

The LES is a one way valve. Its task is to separate the esophagus from the stomach and decides on the food or liquid which enters the stomach. If the sphincter doesn't close properly it becomes over-relaxed. This causes the liquid, food and acid to back up into your esophagus, causing heartburn.

As the research is conflicting, you may want to just try it yourself and see if it really helps you or not.

❖ Aloe Vera Juice

This may not be a tea but aloe vera could be taken in liquid form. Aloe vera juice is made from the gel found in the aloe vera leaves and help to sooth your digestive system and protect against ulcers. In its topical form, it could be used for sunburn, cuts and scalds.

****

There are many herbs and plants which could be made into herbal teas that have various benefits. This simple list should give you a rough idea that could help with your heartburn condition.

Effective Home Remedies For Heartburn

According to my experience, there are more and more people who look to use home remedies to treat heartburn. Check Resource 2 at the back of this book to discover how you can use natural resources to heal heartburn easily and quickly.

Using home remedies can easily heal the heartburn disorder that you are suffering from and improve your overall physical health. Even many Western medical professionals are realizing the incredible effectiveness of the various home treatments.

The discomfort which arise from heartburn attacks are normally described as painful burning sensations which arise from the stomach to the middle of your chest. In more serious cases, it results in esophagus injuries.

Luckily, by opting to make a change in your diet plan, you can easily get rid of heartburn disease. To start, simply trim the number of meals you take to more frequent but smaller portions to ensure that the food you eat get enough time to digest.

Those who look to cure their heartburn might be surprised to find that the natural cures could be easily found in your everyday meals, liquids and herbs.

You could easily begin your natural reflux remedy by including some indigestion foods in your diet which are soft and moist. They are easily and quickly digested.

Foods which are soft could easily flow into your stomach. This allows your esophagus or sphincter to initiate the healing. Keeping away from hard and crunchy food is also important for heartburn patients as it would worsen the problem over time.

Drinking plenty of water is also very important as it helps to keep your LES muscle flap firmly closed over your stomach and this tight seal would prevent stomach acid from flowing into the esophagus. Besides that, water also acts a quick reproduction of tissue cells.

Few people know that honey is an incredible natural home remedy for heartburn. As the problem of heartburns is caused due to your tissues damaging at your esophagus and sphincter, having three spoons of honey each day help repair those tissues.

Apple cider vinegar also acts as a great cure for heartburn. It may taste awful, but it has been proven that if you take just one spoon of it, it could greatly improve your acid levels and food digestion. To make it taste better, you can add some water and honey.

If you are looking for a quicker form of relief, you can have a simple solution of a glass of water, a tablespoon of cumin seeds, coriander juice and a pinch of salt. Besides that, taking carrot juice, coconut water and chewing basil leaves could also help get rid of heartburns.

Home remedies are certainly something you should consider if you don't want to pay excessively for medical prescriptions.

Not only do they result in many side-effects, they could also worsen your condition over time if taken wrongly. If you want a cheaper but slower alternative, home remedies are certainly the way.

Check out this link to find out more about natural cure for heartburns...

http://naturalheartburn.wellbeingvalley.com/

DEALING WITH HEARTBURNS DURING PREGNANCY

As mentioned in earlier chapters, it is very common for pregnant women to suffer from heartburns during the final trimester of their pregnancy.

As the baby grows larger, it would start to put more pressure on the stomach, which inevitably results in the stomach acid flowing back into the esophagus. This causes a burning sensation under the sternum and breastbone, which creates the heartburn problem.

It needs to be clear that heartburns during pregnancy has no side effects on the baby. Besides that, the symptoms of the mother would also vanish when the infant is born. However, before that, the suffering could be incredibly uncomfortable.

In this chapter, I would share some ways in which you can use to get relief. This includes:

➢ **Avoid certain foods** which trigger or activate distress on your gastrointestinal. This includes caffeine, alcohol, chocolates, spicy food, acidic foods and other highly seasoned foods. Acidic foods include mustard, citrus fruits, vinegar or mint products.

➢ As said in the previous chapters, you should **look to take smaller but more frequent portions of meals**. This is similar to most heartburn situations.

➢ **Don't drink too much water when you are eating**. This would cause your stomach distension which triggers your heartburn even further.

➢ **Sleep over additional pillows** as this would elevate the upper body. This would ward off the stomach acid from rising to the chest.

- **Don't wear clothes which are too tight**. This is especially for clothes which emphasises the waist or tummy as it would result in heartburns. Instead, wear looser and more comfortable clothing.
- **If you are smoker**, quit it straight away.
- **Don't lie down or sleep immediately after meals**. The best practice is to go to bed at least three to four hours after eating. This would give your body enough time to digest your food before you sleep.
- **Develop a healthier posture**, and it could help reduce the discomfort in your body to a greater extent. You

should also stand and sit straight. If you bend your knees instead of your waist while picking things up, it would greatly reduce the pressure on your ever-growing tummy.

➢ **Herbal tea** would also help provide relief. Similar to most other heartburn conditions.

From this list, it could be clear that most of the relief for heartburn pregnancy is the same with normal heartburn solutions.

As you follow all these tips and suggestions, you would enjoy a more relaxed and comfortable pregnancy.

This would reduce the pain that you have from heartburn.

HOW HEARTBURN IS CONNECTED TO ARTHRITIS

If you have heartburn symptoms for more than three times in a single week and for a persistent period for three weeks, it is deemed to be chronic heartburn.

Someone who is suffering from persistent heartburn would need to find out the reasons why. This may be because of a recent increased consumption of alcohol, increased stress and intake of certain medication.

If someone has a confirmed chronic heartburn, there would need to be a substantial change in his or her diet. Besides that, a lifestyle change if also required. If you have done all the change but the problem still persists, it could be an indication of other medical problem.

In that case, it is important that you be aware of the reason for someone using natural remedies or certain self-treatment methods to fight the chronic heartburn. This is because certain remedies are simply used to cover the symptoms of more severe problems.

Most of the time, the flow of acid and content into the esophagus from the stomach would cause the acid to irritate the sensitive lining of the stomach.

Very often, when someone suffers from chronic heartburn, he has very irregular dietary habits or takes food which is high in acid content. As such, the digestive system would produce excessive acids which cause further heartburn problems.

In these cases, counter medication would combat the burning sensation which disappears immediately after the substance is processed. If the symptoms are persistent over a longer period, it should be diagnosed immediately and treated with the right prescription medication.

Besides that, heartburn could be possible symptoms for other medical conditions like Gastro-Esophageal Reflux Disease (GERD), pregnancy, hiatal hernia and other stomach related disorders.

Medication for the treatment of many health problems could also cause heartburn. The treatment for illnesses like respiratory problems, arthritis, blood pressure and insomnia are known to create heartburn symptoms.

The most common drug to treat arthritis is non-steroidal anti-inflammatory drugs (NSAIDS). Though those heartburn symptoms are common when using NSAIDS, they correlate badly with bleeding on the tract of gastro-intestine.

These gastrointestinal symptoms like bloating stomach or abdominal pain or heartburn are found in patients who use NSAIDS. This would result in increased difficulty in treating arthritis. Besides that, it is incredibly difficult to predict the time period which an arthritis patient is supposed to use NSAIDS.

Always Take Heartburn Seriously

Most people don't take the problem of heartburn seriously enough until it becomes a chronic condition. As such, the results become pretty serious. As such, there are plenty of reasons to take heartburns seriously.

During the preliminary stages, heartburn is more easily cured. Basically, all you need to do is to take an antacid to ensure that the condition is back to normal. If the problem persists, you would need to go for the super-sized bottles of antacid tablets. They provide fast relief but unfortunately, they are only temporary.

Once you start to realize that you need something more effective and go for other over-the-counter medications, you would realize that your condition would still persist.

Most of those medication offer relief of around 12 to 24 hours only. However, you can't rely on them for months or years as there are side effects which could arise.

You may realize that something is going wrong with your body which require medical attention immediately. You now realize that your heartburn problem would have become a scary malady which intensifies in pain and results in long sleepless night.

You have to head to a doctor right away. The moment you experience your first ever heartburn attack in your life, you should already head for a doctor.

The doctor would pass you a list of the food and liquid that you shouldn't be eating. He would also insist that you lose weight if required. This is hard for many people to follow because many people who have heartburn problems are those who don't have healthy lifestyle habits in the first place.

If you don't want something terrible to happen to you, remember to always take heartburn seriously. If this disease isn't treated seriously, it would lead to more chronic diseases.

Remember that once you reach the incurable stage of heartburn, no medication can help you already. As such, start making lifestyle changes immediately to ensure that your digestive system is working well.

THE BEST DIET TO ALLEVIATE HEARTBURNS

In the previous chapters, I have shared about what food you should avoid as heartburns are heavily affected by the food you eat. If you are suffering from heartburns, you could possibly get rid of those symptoms simply by changing your diets. Using prescriptions drugs may be only the final resort.

There are diets that could reduce the heartburn to a manageable level. Many heartburn patients have flare up late in the evenings and it is important to stop eating late at night. Ensure that you have your meals at the appropriate time to ensure that you are able to properly digest your food before you sleep.

The number one food to stop consuming is acidic food. Foods which are high with acidic content are likely to cause an acid reflux and you should also avoid certain drinks. This includes caffeinated beverages, alcohol and even juice to avoid heartburn symptoms.

You also need to avoid foods which have high fat and hot foods as they would stimulate your stomach. These food should be avoided and try to take healthier food which would reduce the heartburn frequency considerably.

Safer foods include pears, bananas and apples. They are generally better than oranges. Besides, it is important to note that grilled, boiled or baked chicken is better compared to fry. Baked, broiled or boiled seafood are also better than fast-food etc.

Those who are overweight should take smaller but more frequent meals to help them lose weight. This sort of diet would increase their metabolic rate and maintain a proper level of blood glucose.

Besides that, if you are having junk food all the time, you should stop taking them. This is because they are more likely to cause frequent heartburn attacks. You should add a lot of fresh fruits and vegetables in your diet.

As you make these simple changes, your digestion and health would improve. This would eventually decrease your susceptibility to heartburn.

THE MAIN FOODS DURING HEARTBURN

In the United States, heartburn and indigestion makes millions of people extremely miserable. If you are someone who has continuous digestive problems, you need to really treat it with care.

There are a number of foods which could easily trigger heartburn as it relaxes the band of muscles at the end of the esophagus so it can keep acid out from the stomach.

- Spicy food. The main food that you should avoid at all cost are spicy food with chilli powder or black pepper. This also includes garlic and raw onions.
- Citrus foods like tomatoes, grapefruits and oranges.
- Fried or fatty food.
- Alcohol
- Caffeinated drinks like coffee, tea, soda

By avoiding these foods, your heartburn can be greatly lessened or avoided completely. To ensure that you have a better digestive system and to minimize an acid reflux, be sure to get a lot of fibre.

You could get them from non-citrus fruits, vegetables and whole grains. Be sure to drink enough fluids throughout to day to help your body absorb important nutrient and lubricate waste.

You should also be careful about the method of cooking. Stay to cooking by steaming or boiling as they are healthier methods.

Drink some herbal chamomile tea after dinner or before your bedtime. This is believed to have a calming effect on your stomach. You should also bear in mind the atmosphere in which you eat them. Try eating in a calm and relaxed atmosphere where there is little to no distraction.

In the mornings, try eating oatmeal as it is high in fibre, low in saturated fats and cholesterol. Combined with skim milk, it gives a great calcium boost throughout the day. You can add some raisins for taste and also some iron nutrients.

If you are looking to take fruits, focus on taking apples and grapes. They are low in cholesterol, saturated fats and sodium. They are a great choice for Vitamin C and fibre.

In short, these are top foods that should or shouldn't be in your diet:

- **Tangy Citrus Fruits** - Fruits like grapefruits, oranges and orange juice are extremely acidic and are food that you should definitely avoid for heartburn. As such they are likely to cause heartburn, especially when you eat them with an empty stomach.

- **Garlic And Onion** - These food are considered very 'adventurous' and should be avoided. Although some people who have had heartburn wouldn't have an effect when taking them, you should try to avoid them.

- **Spicy Food** - Food which are loaded with pepper or other spices can easily trigger heartburn. You can introduce milder version of them whenever you feel fit.

- **Tomatoes** - Tomatoes are highly acidic and highly likely to cause heartburn to those who are prone to eat.

- **Peppermint** - This is actually a heartburn trigger food. However, this is still up for debate. Many doctors think that it is soothing to the tummy while others believe it triggers heartburn. You should avoid this if you have had a rich meal.

- **Food With High Fat Content** - This includes food like cheese, avacadoes and rib. These food press against the stomach and would a major trigger for heartburn.

- **Alcohol** - This is a definite no-no as alcohol mixes badly with many foods you eat. Drinking wine on its own is alright, but mixing it with other food like meat creates a big effect on your stomach.

The most important thing when it comes to heartburn foods is to find out your triggers. Certain foods which are considered a danger may not affect you that much. Even if your favourite food isn't on this list, you shouldn't necessary take them too frequently.

Too much of a certain type of food could easily trigger heartburn. It is often not what you eat, but rather how much you eat.

Therefore, put in the effort to find out the food that triggers your condition. It will go a long way for improving your heartburn condition over the long run.

FINAL NOTES

The reason for heartburns is when there is an excessive stomach acid leakage into your esophagus or lower throat.

To put it in short, acid reflux, or also known as acid flow back, is a medical term used to describe the situation when the stomach acid flows back from the stomach to the esophagus.

It is a serious digestive disorder which would disrupt the life of the sufferer. If experienced frequently, it would greatly affect the patients' life and be very hard to endure.

This is a pain which is burning and starts from the back of your breastbone and ribs. Then, it radiates towards the throat. This is caused when the acid flows to the esophagus.

Because of the corrosive nature of acid, it would irritate and inflame the esophagus and causes this problem of heartburn. Besides, it varies from mild and irregular to serious and chronic.

If you are suffering from this disorder, consult a doctor immediately. Don't wait until your condition gets serious as it would be way more difficult to cure if your condition gets worst.

By implementing dietary changes and lifestyle changes, you could get rid of heartburn symptoms over time.

If your case of heartburn symptoms occurs more than three times in a single week, it is a sign that your case is very serious. In that case, seek medical assistance immediately.

Good luck with this condition. I wish you the best of health.

RESOURCE 1 - HEARTBURN NO MORE

The free video that this course gives is more than enough for you to know more about heartburn!

Medical Researcher, Nutritionist, Health Consultant and Former Acid Reflux Sufferer Teaches You How To:

- **Permanently Cure Your Acid Reflux Within 2 Months**
- Gain Permanent Relief From Heartburn In 48 Hours!
- **Eliminate Your Chest Pain and Burning Sensation**

- Get Rid of Burping, Belching and Flatulence
- **Dramatically Enhance Digestive and Intestinal Health and Achieve Lasting Freedom From Most Digestive Disorders**
- Get a Peaceful Night Sleep! No More Pain! No More Sleepless Nights! No More Bed-Wedge Pillows!
- **Eliminate the risk of cancer, high blood pressure and Alzheimer's from prescription medications!**
- Save thousands of dollars in prescription medications, over the counters, doctor visits or surgery!
- **Restore Your Energy Levels and Improve The Quality Of Your Life Dramatically...Guaranteed!**

Get it here immediately...

http://heartburnnomore.wellbeingvalley.com/

RESOURCE 2 - NATURAL HEARTBURN CURE

This is an invaluable book that you can use to cure your heartburn problem easily through the use of natural methods.

You don't have to buy any medications. Only pure natural ingredients, which are cheap... Dirt cheap.

Get it here...

http://naturalheartburn.wellbeingvalley.com/